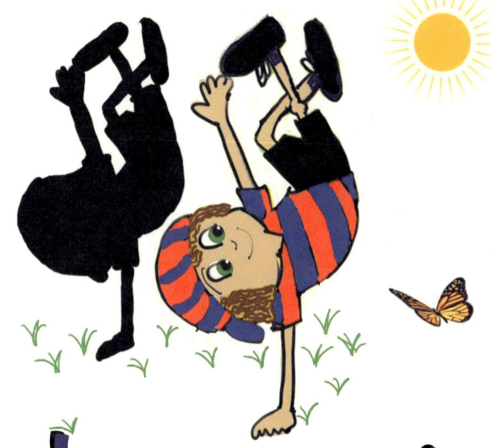

Shadow Dancing

Colleen Guanciale

© 2023 COLLEEN GUANCIALE All rights reserved.

No part of this publication may be reproduced, distributed, or transmitted in any form or by any means, including photocopying, recording, or other electronic or mechanical methods, without the prior written permission of the publisher, except in the case of brief quotations embodied in critical reviews and certain other noncommercial uses permitted by copyright law.

ISBN 978-1-66789-331-0

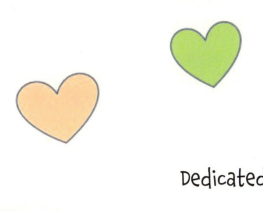

Dedicated to my family—the joy of my life.

My parents, Edward and Dorothy Kamis,
who always looked out for my best interests.

My husband, Christopher Guanciale,
who encouraged me in my projects.

My children, Michael and Kathleen Guanciale,
who always supported me.

My grandchildren, Jayde and Dylan Clift, and Kylie Guanciale,
who are characters in my book.

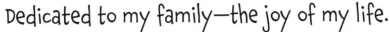

Special thanks to Deneen Watson of St. Mary's Elementary School, Robin Cottrill and CeCe of Silver Lake Pre-School, Ford City, Pa Public Library, Penny Fulton, and all the others who bought and shared my book. It truly is appreciated.

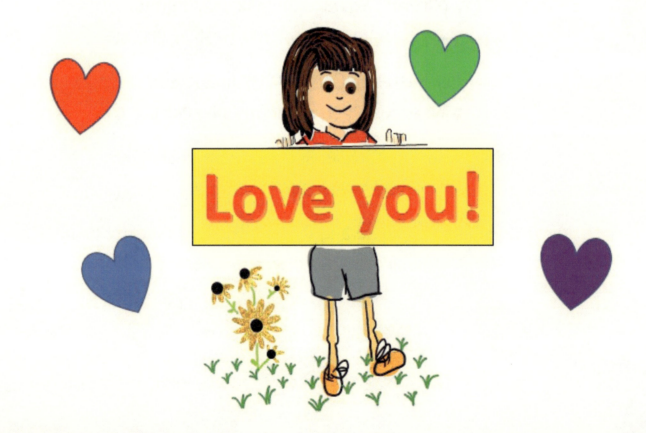

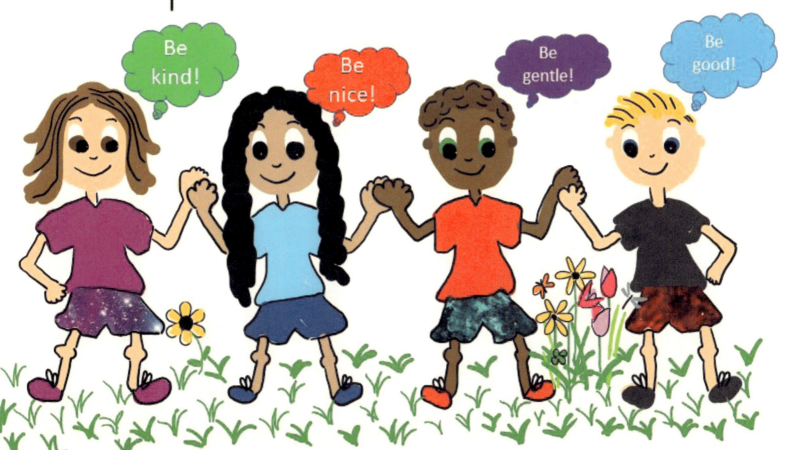

Jayde, Dylan, Kylie, and Joey are going to play a game called "Shadow Dancing." The rules are simple. You shadow their moves.

Shadow dancing is so much fun!

Be my shadow and jump like a rabbit.

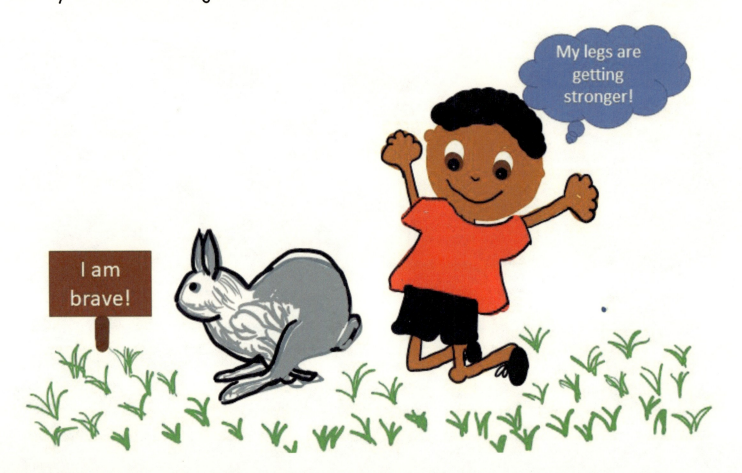

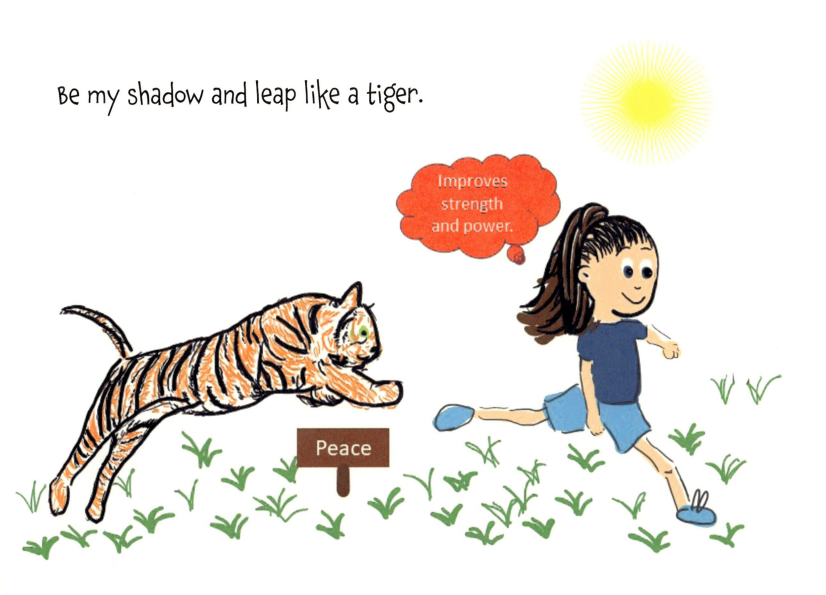

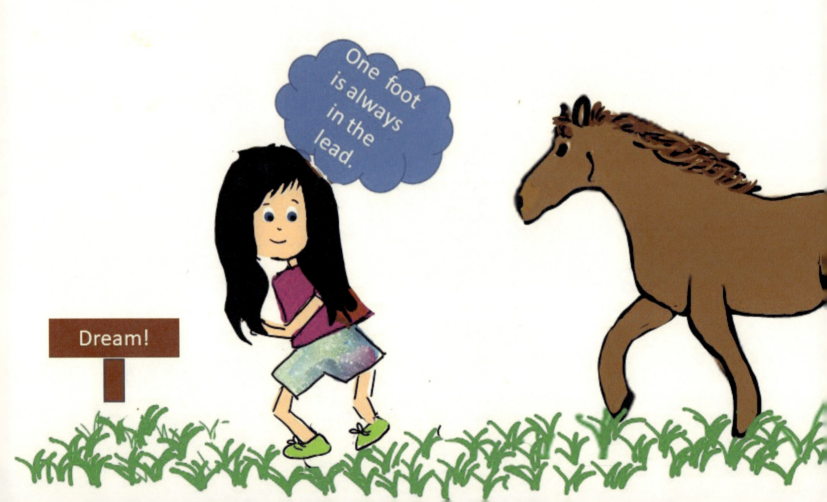

Be my shadow and shake your body like a dog after a bath.
(Head, shoulders, knees, and toes.)

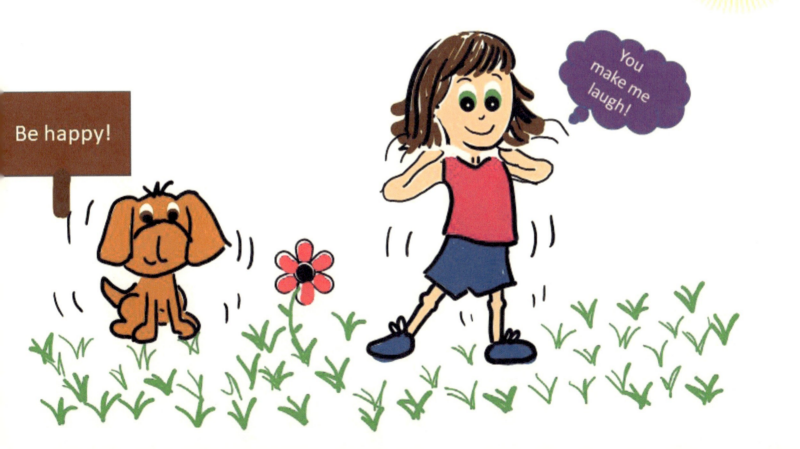

Be my shadow, and leap and ribbit like a frog.
Once you leap like a frog, can you beat your own distance?

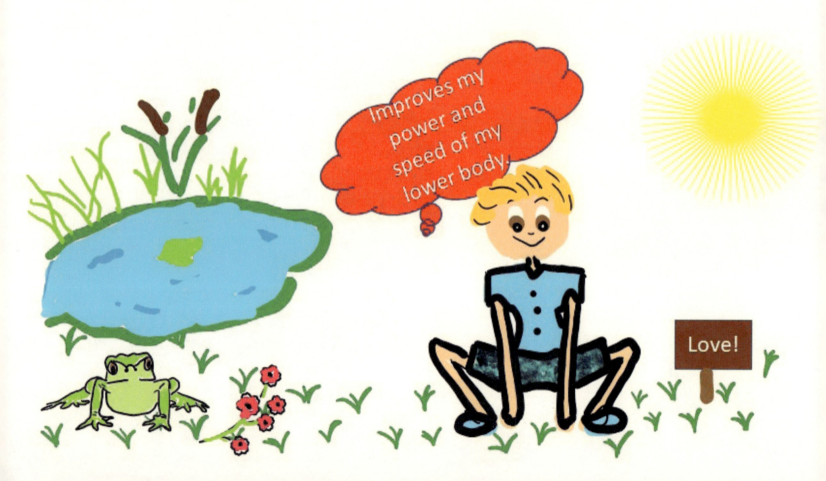

Be my shadow and do the crab walk.

Go forward and backward.

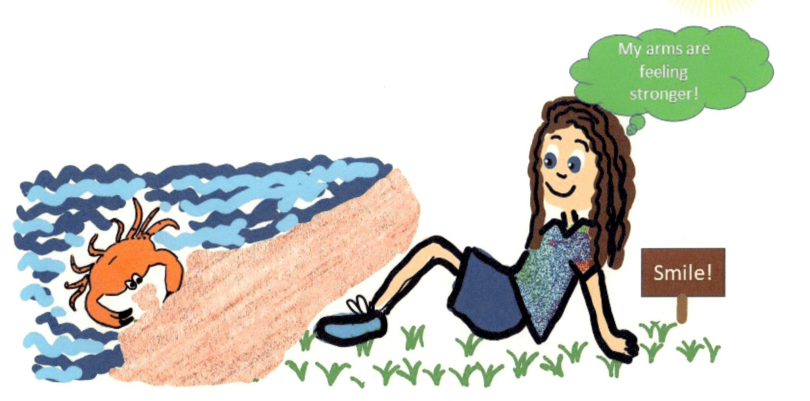

Shadow Dancing is so much fun!

Be my shadow and move like a crocodile.

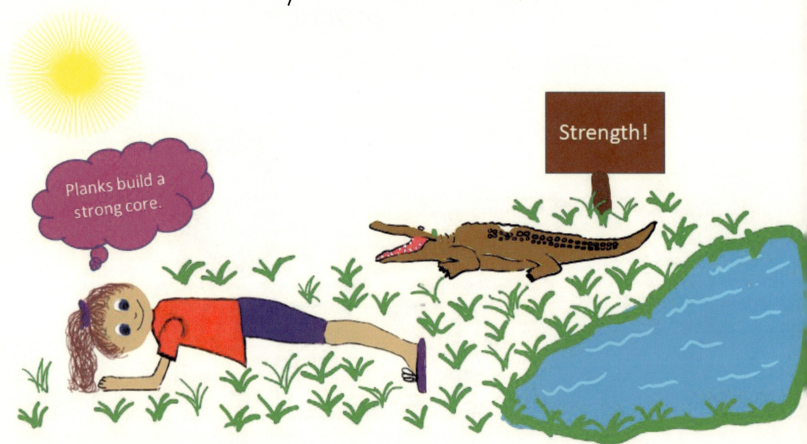

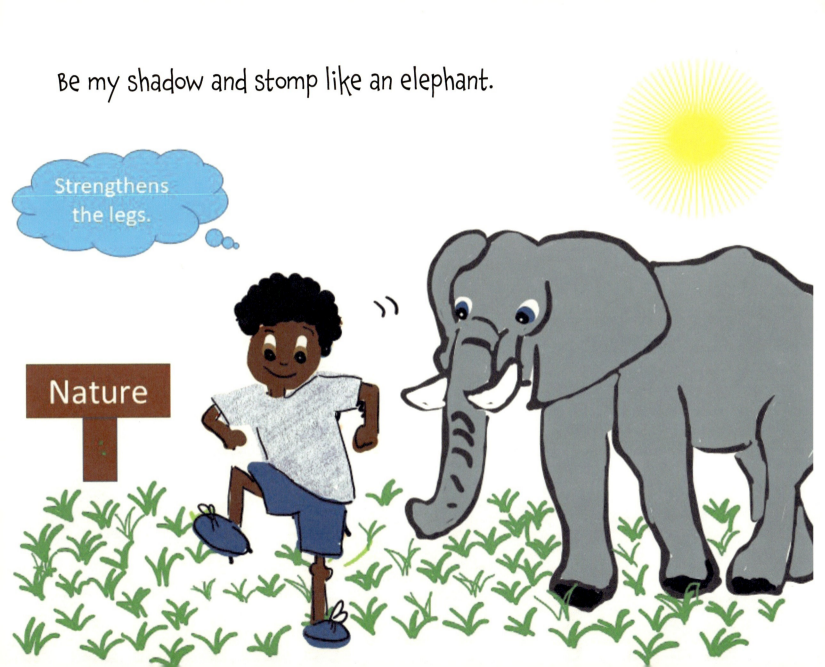

Shadow dancing is so much fun!

Be my shadow and walk like a bear.

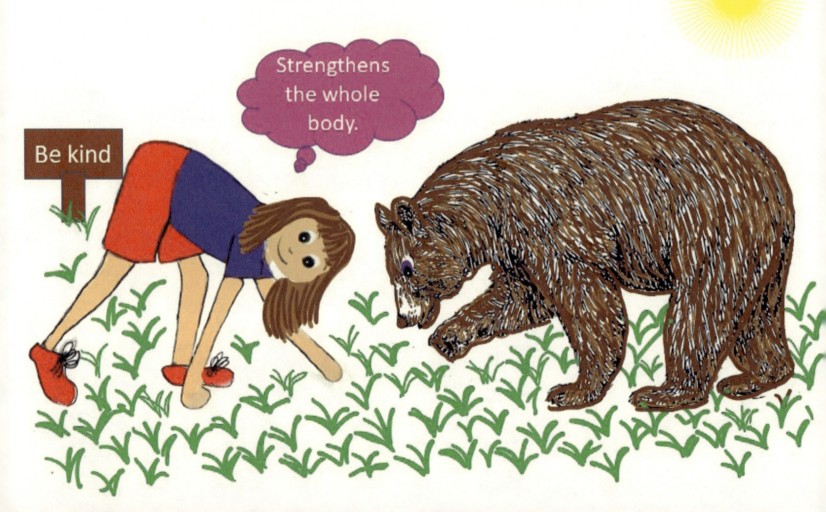

Be my shadow and slither like a snake.

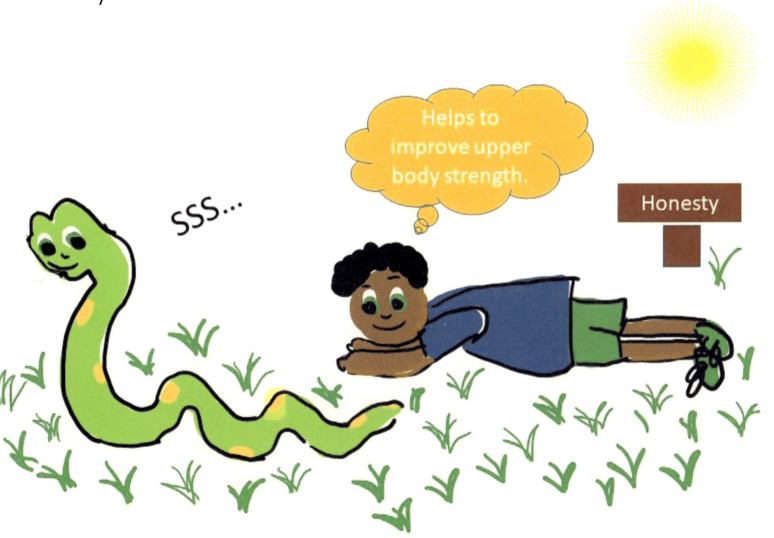

Be my shadow and walk and bark like a seal.
(A moving plank.)

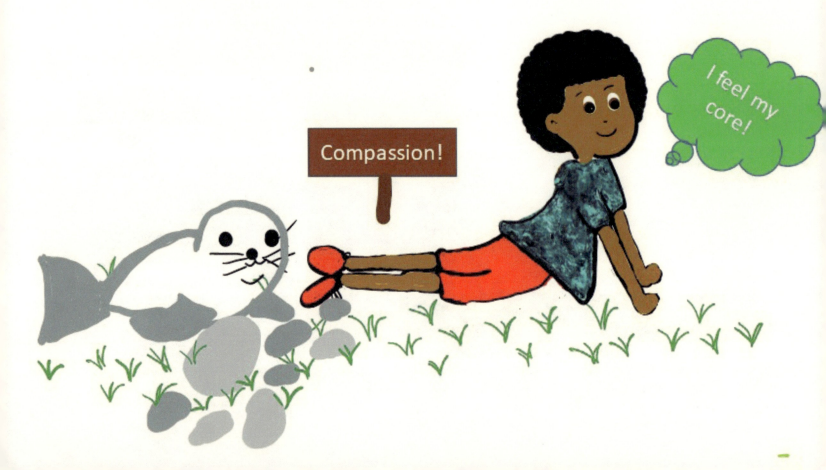

Be my shadow and stand like a flamingo.

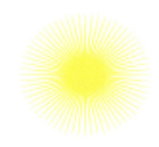

How long can you balance on one leg?

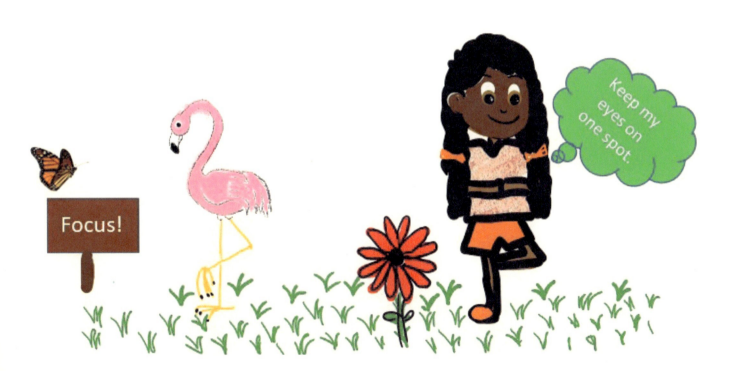

Sit with the bottoms of your feet together; be my shadow, and flap your legs like a butterfly.

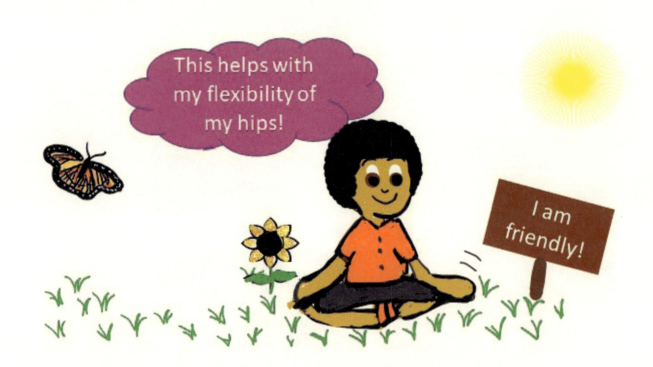

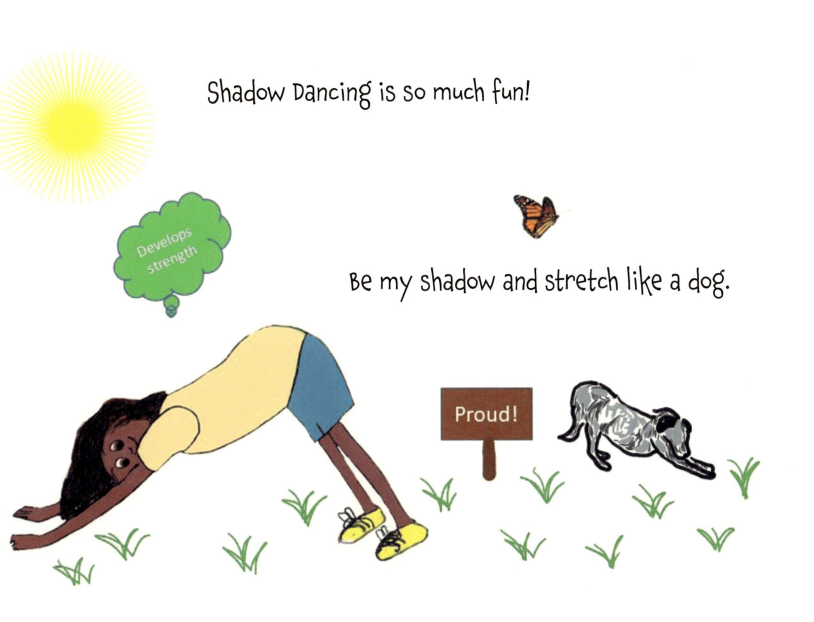

Be my shadow and stretch like a cat.

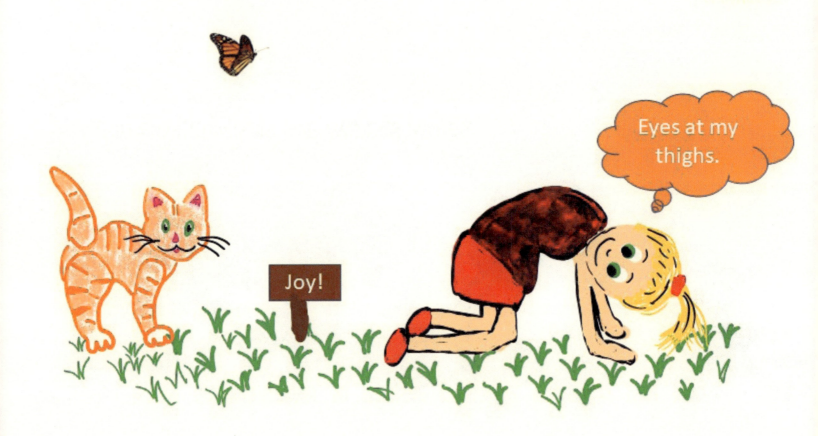

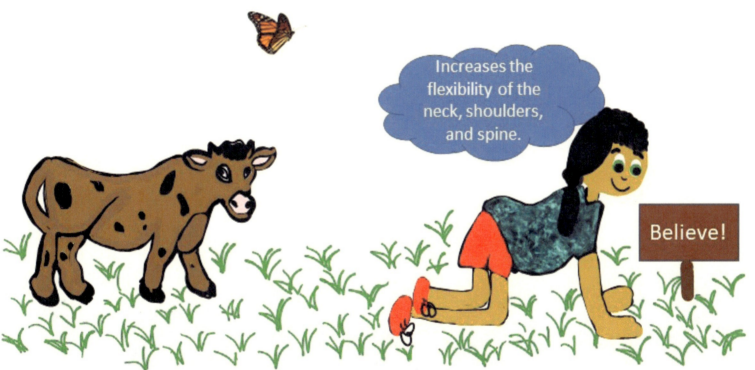

Be my shadow and stretch like a cow.

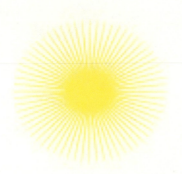

Be my shadow and lie on your back like an upside-down bug.

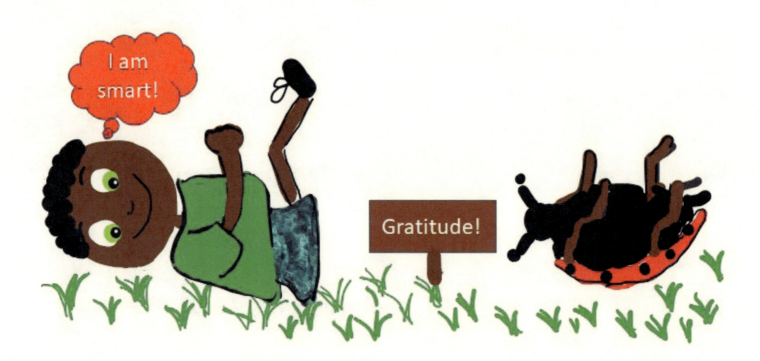

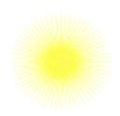
Be my shadow, and lie on your back and relax like a kitten. Stretch.

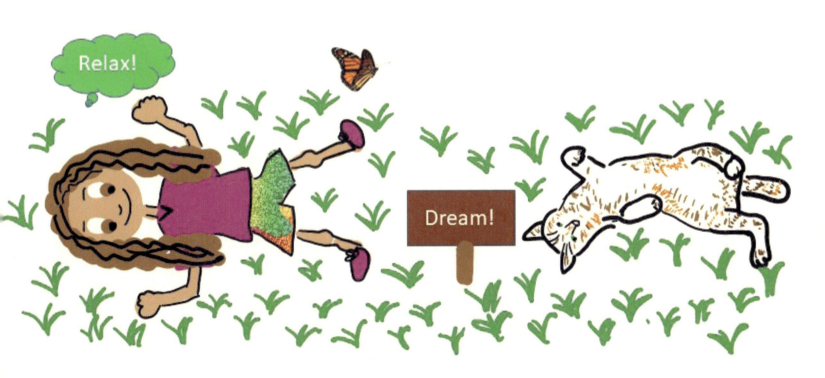

We loved playing Shadow Dancing!

What other animals' shadow would you like to be?

 # The End.

May you be happy.

May you be healthy.

May you always feel like you belong.

Colleen Guanciale is a retired health and physical education teacher. Colleen taught elementary physical education for thirty-four years. She has a B.S. Degree in health and physical education for K-12 curriculum. She is also certified in ACE fitness.

Colleen was always interested in physical activity. In high school, she played basketball. She was the captain of her team and voted the most athletic by her high school peers.

She continued her athletic career in college, where she played college judo. Her accomplishments included being ranked first in Eastern Judo and second in the Nationals. Her team was ranked first in all four years of college.

Colleen loved teaching. She ran the gymnastics, chess, cup stacking, tennis, and boxing clubs for her students. She coached basketball, volleyball, and cheerleading.

In Colleen's leisure time, she enjoys reading, yoga, boxing, dance hit, biking, and being with friends and family.